Alzheimer's Disease:

A Potential $1.1 Trillion Call For Innovative Financial Products and Meaningful Tax Reform

Budd J. Hallberg

authorHOUSE®

AuthorHouse™
1663 Liberty Drive
Bloomington, IN 47403
www.authorhouse.com
Phone: 1 (800) 839-8640

Published by AuthorHouse 12/07/2015

ISBN: 978-1-5049-6131-8 (sc)
ISBN: 978-1-5049-6140-0 (e)

Library of Congress Control Number: 2015918696

Print information available on the last page.

This book is dedicated to the family caregivers of those who struggle daily with Alzheimer's disease. Net proceeds from this text will be given to organizations that conduct research involving Alzheimer's and related disorders.

CONTENTS

ACKNOWLEDGMENTS

*True friendship is like sound health, the value of it
is seldom known until it be lost.*
 -Charles Caleb Colton (1780-1832)

The findings and ideas presented in this book are the result of extraordinary contributions made by friends and colleagues.

I extend thanks to Mary Furlong, M.A. (University of Iowa) who reviewed the manuscript for political theory application and potential unintended consequences.

I owe a debt of gratitude to V. Bruce Hirshauer, Ph.D. (Johns Hopkins University) for reviewing the text and providing me valuable insights and criticism.

I take pleasure in noting Nicole Hummel, B.S. (Juniata College) for the many contributions she made regarding the mechanics and workings of Centers of Excellence which provide for the care, safety and well-being of Alzheimer's patients.

I am most appreciative to Tom Joyce, Ph.D. (Georgetown University) for his comments regarding ethics in business and the moral obligations of lawmakers to do the right thing for their constituents.

I acknowledge Cynthia A. Leggett, M.B.A. (Alvernia University) for her invaluable research into stress associated with the duties and responsibilities of caregiving, and how this has serious psychological and physical impacts on caregiver's health.

I am much obliged to Raymond C. Speciale, Esq., CPA, professor of law and accounting at Mount Saint Mary's University in Emmitsburg, Maryland. His views regarding meaningful tax reform were helpful.

I am fortunate for the academic scholarship provided by Haney Wahba, M.D. (Cairo University Medical School and Post Doctorial training: University of Pittsburgh Medical Center) and his excellent analysis of the serious problems Alzheimer's disease presents not only to the United States, but the world population as a whole.

I am beholden to my former Wall Street colleague Scott Wakefield, A.B. (Yale University) for his expertise in developing new financial products. His encouragement to forge ahead was greatly appreciated.

Finally, I would like to express my gratitude to the many Alzheimer's patients I have met and the wonderful medical personnel who care for them.

PREFACE

The influenza epidemic of 1918-1919 was one of the most devastating scourges in history, killing over 20 million people worldwide. Some recent studies suggest more than 50 million people may have perished from the Spanish Flu. In the United States over 500,000 Americans are believed to have died before the pandemic subsided.[1]

Today, five million Americans suffer from Alzheimer's disease.[2] It is the third leading cause of non-accidental death "behind heart disease and cancer."[3] The medical cost associated with Alzheimer's disease is reported to be $215 billion.[4]

Because of an increasingly aging population, by 2050 the number of people in the United States with Alzheimer's disease is expected to "nearly triple to 13.8 million people."[5] "Unless something's done, the cost is expected to approach $1.1 trillion."[6]

The evidence is convincing. Alzheimer's disease and related disorders are the most serious of healthcare matters in the nation's history.

---

[1] Morens, David M. and Fauci, Anthony S. The 1918 Influenza Pandemic: Insights for the 21st Century. Oxford: The Journal of Infectectous Diseases. Volume 195, Issue 7, pp. 1018-1028, 2007.

[2] National Institute on Aging. Fact Sheet; 2014:1.

[3] Neurology: 2014; 82(12): 1045-50.

[4] National Institute of Health. NIH-supported study finds U.S. dementia care costs as high as $215 billion in 2010; April 3, 2013.

[5] Alzheimer's Association. Alzheimer's Disease Facts and Figures 2015.

[6] Ibid.

The purpose of this essay is to inform the general public about this overwhelming medical crisis facing America today. The goal is to mobilize all Americans to action, thereby causing legal, financial professionals and lawmakers to come together and seek meaningful solutions to this catastrophic problem – Alzheimer's disease.

The objective is to find innovative ways to provide financial relief to designated primary caregivers and centers of excellence for Alzheimer's patients.[7] Action must be taken now and not postponed, for tomorrow is not promised.

---

[7]   Pennsylvania State Plan on Alzheimer's Disease and Related Disorders. Recommendation No. 2. February 7, 2014.

INTRODUCTION

Alzheimer's disease is complex and debilitating. There is no cure for this illness.[8] Once a person has been diagnosed with it, they have been given a death sentence.

The text begins with a discussion about Alzheimer's disease and related disorders. It talks about what the disease is, who discovered it and when. The discourse then focuses on family caregivers, the personal and financial demands made on them, burnout and where they might go to obtain further information on how best to cope with this life changing experience.

The discussion then turns to those medical facilities that provide services to Alzheimer's patients when they come to find they are in need of constant care. In this book, these medical facilities are called *Centers of Excellence for Alzheimer's Disease*. They are wonderful institutions staffed with capable persons who provide for the care, safety and well-being of their residents twenty-four hours a day, seven days a week. This care does not come cheap. It is very expensive and it's that issue which is at the heart of this text.

Next, there is a peek inside The National Alzheimer's Project Act of 2011 and how it places a responsibility on the fifty states in developing comprehensive Alzheimer's disease patient care programs. Studies reveal that the states are not able to assume this task.

---

[8]   Kandel, Eric R., Schwartz, James H., Jessell, Thomas M., Siegelbaum, Steven A. and Hudspeth, A.J. (ed.). *Principles of Neural Science.* New York: McGraw-Medical, 2013, p. 1342.

Nearly all fifty states are in dire financial straits. None of them are administrative or financially equipped to develop and manage an effective Alzheimer's disease and related disorder program.

At the present time, the medical insurance industry is not prepared to meet the financial challenges associated with Alzheimer's disease. Those companies who provide health coverage to the public are of little help. Most are in a merger and acquisition mode and ignore developing Alzheimer's disease health plans for policy holders.

Two new financial products are introduced in chapter six. If these products are carefully designed and marketed, they could help mitigate the ballooning costs associated with Alzheimer's disease and related disorders. Chapter seven discusses a number of ways to enact meaningful tax reform legislation that would help caregivers deal with the financial burden they face each day. Where applicable, this chapter also addresses healthcare facility property tax relief and other amenities that could reduce the cost of healthcare for AD patients.

Concluding remarks summarize many of the wonderful accomplishments made by research at a number of colleges and universities as well as efforts being made by a number of the major pharmaceutical companies which focus on the treatment and hopeful cure for Alzheimer's disease. While these activities are noble and worthy of recognition, for the most part, they are long-range programs. Immediate relief is needed now for caregivers and institutions that provide services for the well-being and safety of those stricken with AD, and that's what this book is about.

The Epilogue points out that the Alzheimer's disease crisis in America is a global pandemic. Governments around the world are beginning to look at this medical issue first, as an *Ethical* matter, then how the medical industry views itself, the notion of self-governance, and as a *Moral Obligation* they have to their citizenry. Final remarks call for a transparent debate among medical industry chiefs and lawmakers to come to a consensus as to how best resolve the current medical crisis associated with ADRD.

CHAPTER ONE

ALZHEIMER'S DISEASE

The tragedy of life is what dies inside a man while he lives.
-Albert Schweitzer

What is Alzheimer's disease?

"Alzheimer's disease is a form of progressive mental deterioration due to generalized degeneration of the brain, occurring in middle or old age."[9]

Other dementias include: vascular dementia, mixed dementia, dementia with Lewy Bodies, Parkinson's disease dementia, Frontotemporal dementia, Creuzfeldt-Jacob dementia, Normal Pressure Hydrocephalus, Huntington's disease, Wernicke-Korsakoff

---

[9] Pearsall, Judy. *The Concise Oxford Dictionary.* Oxford: Oxford University Press, 1999, p. 40.
"A substantial cognitive decline from a previous level of performance in one or more of the domains outlined above based on the concerns of the individual, a knowledgeable informant, or the clinician; and a decline in neurocognitive performance, typically involving test performance in the range of two or more standard deviations below appropriate norms (i.e., below the third percentile) on formal testing or equivalent clinical evaluation."
American Psychiatric Association. *Diagnostic and Statistical Manual of Mental Disorders.* 5th ed. Arlington, VA:
American Psychiatric Publishing; 2013:section 2.

Syndrome and Mild Cognitive Impairment. These are commonly referred to as "related dementias."

Alzheimer's disease (AD, or, the disease) and related disorders (RD) are characterized by loss of memory to the point so severe that it interferes with a person's activities associated with daily living. Early signs common to AD are the inability to remember even simple things. Reasoning is visibly impaired and there is little interest in planning for things.

When AD was first discovered.

The disease was discovered in 1906 by Alois Alzheimer, a German psychiatrist, while performing an autopsy on a former patient. During the procedure, Alzheimer observed a number of pathological conditions including: presence of neurofibrillary tangles, amyloid plaques and atrophy.[10] These factors were persuasive enough to cause a diagnosis of senile dementia which today is called Alzheimer's disease.

Types of Alzheimer's disease.

There are three types of AD. They are: 1) Early-onset Alzheimer's, 2) Late-onset Alzheimer's and 3) Familial Alzheimer's Disease (FAD).

Early-onset Alzheimer's happens to people who are younger than 65. Often, they're in their 40s or 50s when they're diagnosed with the disease. It's rare - less than 10% of all people with AD have early-onset. People with *Down Syndrome* have a higher risk for it, since they tend to age faster.

Scientists have found a few ways in which Early-onset AD is different from other types of the disease. People who have it tend to have more of the brain changes that are linked with AD. The

---

[10]   Kandel, pp. 1335-1340.

Early-onset form also appears to be linked with a defect in a specific part of a person's DNAS: chromosome 14. A form of muscle twitching and spasm, called mycoclonus, is also more common in Early-onset AD.

Late-onset Alzheimer's is the most common form of the disease, which happens to people age 65 and older. It may or may not run in families. So far, researchers haven't found a particular gene that causes it. No one knows for sure why some people get it and others don't.

Familial Alzheimer's Disease is a form of AD that doctors know for certain is linked to genes. In families that are affected, members of at least two generations have had the disease. FAD makes up less than 1% of all cases of AD. People who have it start showing signs very early on, often in their 40s.[11]

Alzheimer's Disease Can Be Diagnosed Well but Available Treatments Are Poor.[12]

Diagnosing AD in the early stages is a difficult process. It is hard to distinguish between the onset of AD and the typical decline often associated with aging in general. "In the 1970s diagnostic error rates were approximately 30%, as judged by best objective measure ..."[13] While progress is being made on a number of fronts, the pace is slow. Today, there is no cure for AD. Once diagnosed with the disease, the patient's condition is terminal.

The Alzheimer's Association has identified ten warning signs of AD. They are: 1) memory loss that affects job skills, 2) difficulty performing familiar tasks, 3) problems with language, 4) disorientation of time and place, 5) poor or decreased judgment, 6)

---

[11] WebMD Medical Reference. SOURCE: Alzheimer's Association. Reviewed by: Neil Lava, MD on July 10, 2014.

[12] Kandel, p. 1341.

[13] Ibid.

problems with abstract thinking, 7) misplacing things, 8) changes in mood or behavior, 9) changes in personality and 10) loss of initiative.[14]

Common themes for older caregivers.

Once a family member has been diagnosed with AD, a number of factors begin to resonate with the primary caregiver and close family members left behind to care for that person. Those themes include: "1) lack of information, especially at a time of diagnosis, 2) profound *sense of **Loss*** with further diagnosis, 3) fear about (the) future - including financial fears, 4) difficulty formulating long-term plan(s), 5) struggle to access community based coordinated care, 6) difficulty partnering with (the) medical community, 7) overwhelmed by demands of caregiving, 8) isolation and abandonment and 9) end of life issues."[15]

Take the twelve minute journey into the world of a person afflicted with Alzheimer's disease.

You can experience for yourself, the dark world of a person who has been diagnosed with Alzheimer's disease.[16] It is a world of *deficit, decline* and *death*.[17] Alzheimer's disease robs a person of everything that's of value to them. It takes away one's past through the loss of memory; important and meaningful relationships disappear and a

---

[14] Alzheimer's Association.

[15] Hoffman, David. Alzheimer's Disease Caregiver Support Initiative. *Advisory Council on Alzheimer's Research, Care, and Services.* US Department of Health and Human Services, 200 Independence Avenue, SW, Washington, DC. July 27, 2015.
Glatzer, Richard and Westmorland, Wash. *Still Alice.* Killer Films. DVD. December 5, 2014. Appendix C.

[16] http://youtu.be/LL Gq7She-Y.

[17] Wells, Samuel. Dementia and resurrection. London: Christian Century, April 1, 2015, p. 33.

person's dignity and self-esteem diminish, and then finally disappear. There is a constant struggle to 'hold on' – to avoid decline, but the battle is futile.[18] Death will eventually unlock the doors to this prison.

Caregiver Burnout.

Caregivers experience a great deal of stress as they try to deal with the many problems associated with AD. Burnout is common and leads to the need to make substantial readjustments to their lives.[19]

How people respond to stress varies.[20] Some are able to cope more effectively than others. Coping falls into two categories: 1) problem-focused and 2) emotion-focused.[21] Those persons who experience difficulty in managing stress will oftentimes act out and abuse a loved one suffering from ADRD. In these instances, both caregiver and AD patient are severely harmed.[22]

Comprehensive and meaningful ADRD educational materials and training programs are available to Caregivers.

There are a number of organizations that provide valuable information to the public in regard to ADRD as well as training programs for family caregivers. Available materials often help AD patients and their caregivers to understand better the nature of the disease and the financial challenges which lie ahead. A partial list of those organizations can be found in Appendix A.

---

[18]   Ibid.

[19]   Nolan-Hoeksema, Susan, Fredrickson, Barbara L., Loftus, Geoffrey R., and Lutz, Christel. *Atkinson & Hilgard's Introduction to Psychology.* Andover: Cengage Learning, 2014, p. 472.

[20]   Reinhard, Susan C., Feinberg, Lynn Friss, Choula, Rita and Houser, Ari. Valuing the Invaluable: 2015 Update. AARP Public Policy Institute, July 2015, p. 7.

[21]   Nolan-Hoeksema, p. 487.

[22]   Ibid, p. 481.

CHAPTER TWO

CENTERS OF EXCELLENCE FOR ALZHEIMER'S DISEASE

Care more for the individual patient than for the special features of the disease.

-Sir William Osler

O nce a person is diagnosed with AD, there will come a time they will be in need of constant professional care. Institutions that provide this service are oftentimes referred to as healthcare centers, AD care facilities – here they are called Centers of Excellence for Alzheimer's Disease (Centers of Excellence, or CoE).[23]

Each state has a number of CoEs which operate within their borders. Some CoEs are state government operated; others function as profit-making organizations while many operate as non-profit entities. A number of CoEs are anchored to a particular religious organization. CoEs operate under federal and state regulation.

Regardless of the core structure, families of a CoE resident can feel comfortable that their family member is being well-cared for by qualified personnel and living in a state of the art facility. That said quality care doesn't come cheap. Depending on the services provided

---

[23]   Formerly known as Alzheimer's Disease Assistance Centers.
Also; healthcare quarters, assisted living facility, etc.
Hoffman, David. <u>Alzheimer's Disease Caregiver Support Initiative.</u>

and CoE location, care can range from $5,000 - $20,000 a month. In some instances, the cost can be higher.

Centers of Excellence are typically a part of a larger healthcare facility. They are often referred to as a 'Unit of' or a 'Wing' – a place devoted solely to the care of AD patients.

Centers of Excellence are often headed by a Director and have on board a support staff of registered nurses and professionally trained – licensed caregivers. Psychiatrists, neurologists, psychologists and medical doctors are either full-time staff members or immediately available on-call, depending on the size and nature of the CoE.

The Patient Protection and Affordable Care Act (PPACA) was signed into law on March 23, 2010. This law has placed enhanced requirements on CoEs to monitor electronically the care of AD patients on a twenty-four hour, seven days a week basis. This provides an audit trail should something go wrong with a particular AD resident's care.

For both the protection of the CoE and AD residents, it is essential that CoEs have in place a comprehensive set of guidelines in the form of a written Policy and Procedures Manual (P&P Manual, Policy Manual, the manual). At a minimum, the manual should have a *Mission Statement* including the CoE's *Goals, and Objectives* of operations. The Policy Manual should articulate the organization's policy regarding *Resident Confidentiality* and its philosophy concerning *Principles of Medical Ethics*.

At a minimum, a CoE's Policy Manual should address the following topics for explanation and provide guidance to all professional and non-professional staff associated with the CoE: 1) certification, licensing requirements and identification 2) resident care, 3) organization and management of the CoE, 4) duties and responsibilities of all job descriptions to be performed by those full-time staff members who comprise the AD unit within the organization, 5) procedures to be used in handling emergencies, 6) continued education and training of professional CoE staff members, 7) code of conduct, 8) professional appearance, attire, 9) types of unacceptable behavior – use of iPhones during duty hours, making loud noise, approved methods when approaching residents, 10) policy on holidays, sick leave and vacation, and 11) security. The manual should address such things as Equal Employment Opportunity (EEO) hiring policy and the establishment of a safe work environment for all employees.[24]

Many CoEs make use of volunteers. The Policy Manual should include a section dealing with such non-employee activities to provide guidance regarding: 1) sign-in procedures, 2) wearing identification badges, 3) dress code, 4) reporting resident accidents and illness, 5) making purchases on behalf of residents, 6) performing first aid on a resident, 7) maintaining good personal hygiene, 8) making telephone calls, or letter writing on behalf of residents, 9) taking residents for trips and walks, 10) general demeanor – smile, 11) communication techniques, and 12) reporting levels – chain-of-command. Centers of Excellence should ensure volunteers have attended a thorough Orientation Program before assuming tasks associated with residents' care.

When selecting a CoE for a family member stricken with AD, caregivers should look to make sure such written Policy Manual is in place.

A typical day in the life of an AD resident at a CoE.

Centers of Excellence have developed a daily structure for AD residents to follow. This procedure allows for residents to be engaged with one another and live as normal a life as possible given their particular set of circumstances. It also provides guidance to professional staff of the CoE as to their duties and responsibilities as stated in their job descriptions. This structure is critical for the safety and well-being of the residents.

---

[24] Reference: Harvard Medical School at: hms.harvard.edu.

A CoE's resident daily schedule often includes specific times for such activities as: 1) breakfast, 2) life skills and discussion, 3) exercise, 4) socializing, 5) storytelling, 6) sing-along, 7) pre-lunch preparation, 8) lunch, 9) quiet time, 10) socializing, 11) exercise, 12) sing-along, 13) word games, 14) pre-dinner preparation, 15) dinner, 16) events, 17) music video, 18) pre-evening preparation and 19) bedtime. A more detailed listing of a resident's daily routine can be found in Appendix B.

AD residents' care, safety and well-being must always come first. To ensure these goals and objectives are achieved, it is critical that states' ADRD programs be focused on their Centers of Excellence. These facilities must be state of the art and staffed by the best professional caregivers in their career field. The work involving residents' care is labor intensive. The cost of running such operations doesn't come cheap. They are expensive and costs are expected to increase over the coming years. State governments need to put themselves in a crisis action mode. They should begin taking action now to ensure that all of the states' CoEs continue long-term operations and are successful.

CHAPTER THREE

THE NATIONAL ALZHEIMER'S PROJECT ACT OF 2011

The legitimate object of government is to do for a community of people whatever they need to have done, but cannot do at all in their separate and individual capacities.
                              -Abraham Lincoln (1809-1865)

C ongress recognized the severity AD presents to the American people. In December 2010, they passed The National Alzheimer's Project Act (Act, or the Act, law, or the law) which was signed into law by President Barrack Obama on January 4, 2011.[25]

The essence of the Act has three parts. First, it places the U.S. Department of Health and Human Services (HHS) in a central administrative role ensuring compliance with the law. Second, it requires the crafting of a National Plan as to how best overcome AD. Third, it makes it quite clear, that recommendations dealing with the costs associated with ADRD don't compromise the integrity of established Medicare and Medicaid programs.

---

[25] Alzheimer's Association.

Specifically, PUBLIC LAW 111-375-JAN. 4, 2011 in part reads:
SEC. 2 THE NATIONAL ALZHEIMER'S PROJECT.

(5) ANNUAL REPORT. –

    (A) an initial evaluation of all federally funded efforts in Alzheimer's research, clinical care, and institutional-, home-, and community-based programs and their outcomes;

    (B) initial recommendations for priority actions to expand, eliminate, coordinate, or condense programs based on the program's performance, mission, and purpose;

    (C) initial recommendations to-

        (i) reduce the financial impact of Alzheimer's on-

            (I) Medicare and other federally funded programs; and
            (II) families living with Alzheimer's disease;

        and

        (ii) improve health outcomes; and

    (D) annually thereafter, an evaluation of the implementation, including outcomes, of the recommendations, including priorities if necessary, through an updated national plan under subsection (d)(2). (sic). Appendix D.

The law is quite clear. Each of the 50 states cannot rely solely on federal government programs like Medicare to fund their ADRD obligations. They are going to have to enact legislation and build internal AD programs to operate within their borders to deal effectively with the costs associated with the care of those afflicted with ADRD. Time is not on the side of state lawmakers. They need to come to terms with this matter and act now.

CHAPTER FOUR

STATES ARE ILL-PREPARED TO DEAL WITH THE ALZHEIMER'S DISEASE CRISIS

Our task now is not to fix the blame for the
the past, but to fix the course for the future.
                                        -John F. Kennedy

While some states are in a better financial position to deal with the coming responsibility to develop and fund a comprehensive ADRD program within their borders, the majority of states are ill-prepared to tackle this job. Nearly all states are debt burdened with financial obligations committed to other programs.

The Study.

A study was made of ten (10) states, or twenty percent (20%) of the nation's composition, to examine: 1) estimates of total numbers of Americans age 65 and older with Alzheimer's by state and the projection change for the period 2015-2025 and 2) how well those states are positioned to develop and financially administer a comprehensive ADRD program. States selected for review were based on demographics (with an emphasis on diversity) and geographical dispersion.

The study included an examination of projections and financial conditions of the following states: 1) Alabama, 2) Arkansas, 3) California, 4) Florida, 5) Illinois, 6) Maine, 7) New York, 8) Texas, 9) Washington and 10) West Virginia.

Projections of Percentage Change 2015-2025.[26]

State	Projected Number w/ Alzheimer's (in thousands)		Percentage Change
	2015	2025	2015-2025
Alabama	87	110	26.4%
Arkansas	53	67	26.4
California	590	840	42.4
Florida	500	720	44.0
Illinois	210	260	23.8
Maine	26	35	34.6
New York	380	460	21.1
Texas	340	490	44.1
Washington	100	140	40.0
West Virginia	36	44	22.2

---

[26]   Alzheimer's Association. Alzheimer's Disease Facts and Figures 2015.

How well are the sample states positioned financially, to meet these future obligations?[27]

Alabama had the 15th worst "Taxpayer Burden" of all 50 states. Each taxpayer's burden was ($13,400).

The state of Arkansas had the 35th best "Taxpayer Burden" of all 50 states. Their debt amounted to ($1,500) per taxpayer. Most of the state's debt is unpaid retirement promises.

California had the 8th worst "Taxpayer Burden" of all 50 states in 2013. Each taxpayer's burden was ($20,900). The money needed to pay its bills had a deficit of $234.6 billion that year.

The state of Florida is sinking in debt. The state owned $59.5 billion in assets and owed $74.3 billion in expenditures. Each taxpayer's share of this financial obligation was ($2,500).

Illinois had the 2nd worst "Taxpayer Burden" of all 50 states in 2013. The burden per taxpayer is a staggering ($45,000) and is 94% of Illinois average income of $48,120.

The state of Maine had the 20th worst "Taxpayer Burden" of all 50 states in 2013. Each taxpayer's burden amounts to ($8,800).

New York did not have enough available assets to cover its debt. Each taxpayer's burden amounted to ($20,700).

On June 9, 2015, the state of Texas released financial data for 2014. Texas owed more than it owned. The state did not have enough available assets to cover its debt. Each taxpayer's burden amounted to ($8,300).

Washington State's bills exceeded its assets. Obligations amounted to $56 billion while available assets were valued at $36 billion. "Truth in Accounting's detailed analysis discovered a total of $15 billion of retirement benefits are owed, but not funded." Taxpayer's Burden was ($8,500).

---

[27] The data source used for the study was 'state data lab' prepared by: Truth in Accounting, 118 North Clinton Street, Suite 206, Chicago, IL 60661. www.truthinaccounting.org.

West Virginia had the 11th worst "Taxpayer Burden" of all 50 states. Obligation per taxpayer was ($13,000). The state did not have enough assets to cover its debt.

The outcome of this sampling of future projected obligations and the financial condition of the twenty percent of states in the United States sampled, holds little hope that states as a whole will be in a financial position to develop comprehensive ADRD programs.

In the near term, Medicare will be looking to: 1) increase policyholder premiums, 2) decrease medical payments for healthcare in general and 3) through the Act, protect what assets Medicare and Medicaid have against an Alzheimer's disease invasion of funds.

It is evident that insurance companies are in a merger and acquisition phase. They are not financially prepared to step up to the plate and do what they need to do to enhance medical coverage for ADRD patient and caregiver costs.

Taxpayers are financially exhausted.

For the most part, the general public is not financially prepared to have their taxes raised to fund another medical program whose unintended consequences have not been clearly defined. Given these circumstances, the states are going to have to look to innovative ways to fund their ADRD programs. Two considerations lawmakers must consider are: 1) developing innovative financial products and 2) enacting meaningful tax reform legislation to meet this national epidemic.

CHAPTER FIVE

MEDICAL INSURANCE COVERAGE OPTIONS ARE LIMITED

A great society is a society in which men of business think greatly of their functions.
-Alfred North Whitehead

The vast majority of working Americans retire at age 65. For many, planning for medical insurance coverage into retirement years is difficult. To include a provision in post-retirement medical coverage for some form of payment should they be stricken with AD is a nightmare.[28] If the retiree has already been diagnosed with the disease prior to retirement, the exercise is futile. Medical insurance coverage for AD is either not available, or if it is, the insurance premium payments are prohibitive.

At the time of retirement, most Americans opt to either: 1) remain in their employer's group health insurance plan or 2) select Medicare. In either case, at present, retirees must purchase some form of supplemental medical insurance to support their major plan of choice. Finding a supplemental plan that would cover ADRD is near impossible. Again, if one is available, the premium to coverage ratio is out of reach for the majority of people.

---

[28] Alzheimer's disease typically makes itself noticeable in people ages 65 and older.

For those afflicted with AD and who are now residents of a CoE their sources of income to pay for their monthly care is typically derived from some combination of the following sources: 1) Social Security Disability, 2) Medicare, 3) a private medical insurance plan and 4) personal family resources. In most instances, family assets pay for the largest amount due for their family member's care. In a matter of time, many families find themselves insolvent.

Medicare rules are complicated.

Medicare has strict enrollment rules. If people miss a deadline such as the 'special enrollment period' they can find themselves without medical coverage for a number of months. For AD patients, the application process to obtain benefits from Medicare and Medicaid is lengthy and complicated.

Retirees who elect to remain with their previous employer's group health insurance plan often find that what was once covered under the plan when they were employed is no longer covered now that they are retired. Coverage has changed. Discovery of this condition comes the hard way – usually when a person files a claim for a particular medical treatment and the "plan rejects their claim."[29]

Double-digit price increases for Medicare Part B premiums are scheduled to come in 2016. "The boost may be 15% of all participants or a whopping 52% for some."[30] So what is a 65 year-old retiree to do in planning for health insurance coverage in their Golden Years?

The Healthcare Insurance Industry is in a state of flux.

A recent article in *The New York Times* entitled "Cigna Rejects an Overture from Anthem" authors Michael J. de la Merced and Reed

---

[29] Kiplinger's Retirement Report. Don't Get Trapped By Medicare Rules. May 2015.

[30] The Kiplinger Letter. Vol. 92, No. 31. July 31, 2015.

Abelson note "The world of American health insurance may soon become even smaller, with the biggest companies seeking to become even bigger."[31] They go on to say that the Affordable Care Act has been a driving force in causing a flurry of merger discussions among major medical insurers, "giving them access to millions of additional customers through state market places."[32] That assumes the state market places are an efficient price discovery mechanism.

First, not all states 'have insurance exchanges."[33] Second, those states that have exchanges sometimes fail to function as an efficient marketplace.

The Vermont Experience.

Vermont lawmakers viewed President Obama's Affordable Care Act as the gateway to a single-payer healthcare plan for all its citizenry. Unexpectedly, the state's online insurance marketplace began to have extensive technical failures causing a 'crisis in confidence' among much of the state's residents. "Despite an eventual cost of up to $200 million in federal funds, Vermont's online marketplace is still not fully functional."[34] The state's experience provides a cautionary tale.

The Insurance Industry is not well positioned.

Right now, insurance companies are in a merger and acquisition phase, presumably to reduce costs and pass those savings on to medical insurance policyholders. There is one key overarching question. Will

---

[31] de la Merced, Michael and Abelson, Reed. Cigna Rejects an Overture From Anthem. *The New York Times.* Section B1. Monday, June 22, 2015.

[32] Ibid.

[33] Forbes, Steve. The Constitution Does It Matter Anymore? *Forbes.* July 20, 2015, p. 13.

[34] Goodnough, Abby. Barely Meeting a Law It Hoped to Transcend. *The New York Times.* Friday, June 5, 2015, pp. A12 and A15.

insurance company consolidation "trickle down to the consumer or wind up in the pocket of shareholders?"[35]

Insurance companies don't appear to be crafting new types of AD medical coverage policies aimed at enhancement of ADRD patient and CoE coverage. This in turn, has not positioned the insurance industry well for assisting the fifty states in meeting their obligations to develop comprehensive ADRD programs.

Lawmakers and insurance company executives must find some common ground, come together now and seek ways to enact legislation which will cause insurance providers to refocus their energies and design new medical policies that will provide some coverage for all AD patients – regardless of time and place in the diagnostic process. This must be a cooperative effort and make it a win-win for the AD patient, CoEs and insurance providers.

---

[35] Sorkin, Andrew Ross. Health Care Law Spurs Merger Talks for Insurers. *The New York Times.* Business Section. June 22,2015, pp. 1 and 5.

CHAPTER SIX

NEW FINANCIAL PRODUCTS

Business has only two functions-marketing and innovation.
-Peter Drucker

The federal debt is worse than you think.

According to a recent study made by Ron Haskins of the Brookings Institution in Washington, DC, the national debt of the United States "ballooned to 78 percent of Gross Domestic Product (GDP) in 2013, almost twice the pre-recession (2008) level.[36] He goes on to say, that although the annual deficit is now declining, it will begin to once again start to increase, and by 2020, "we will once again return to annual deficits above a trillion dollars, thereby once again greatly increasing the national debt."[37] America is not in a financial position to launch a fiscally sound Alzheimer's disease and related disorder program. That is to say,

---

[36] Pearsall. Gross Domestic Product is: the total value of goods produced and services provided in a country during one year.

[37] Haskins, Ron. The federal debt is worse than you think. Washington: Brookings Institution, April 8, 2015, p. 1.

The states are broke and the nation is in financial ruin.

The evidence is persuasive. None of the fifty states are anywhere close to being financially equipped to develop comprehensive ADRD programs now, let alone well on into the year 2050. National, state and local governments are going to have to look at innovative ways to deal with this overwhelming medical problem. If they don't, the outcome will be nothing less than social chaos and whirl.

National government partnerships with the private sector to seek lasting solutions to the ADRD health and financial crisis.

LONDON, March 17, 2015:
"J.P. Morgan today announced that it has been working with the U.K. government to develop a new multi-million pound fund to encourage investment into better treatments for dementia, a condition that affects an estimated 47 million people worldwide. The firm is providing financial advice to the government and support through its knowledge and experience of the healthcare industry to help identify private sector investment. The aim of the Dementia Discovery Fund (the "Fund") is to create an innovative collaboration that will bring together the combined expertise and resources of J. P. Morgan, the U.K. government, national research organizations, and major pharmaceutical companies, including clients of the firm."

A Precedent has been set.

The coming together of the U.K. government and J. P. Morgan in establishing the Dementia Discovery Fund is a clear recognition that governments alone are not going to be able to deal effectively with the ADRD dilemma. They are going to have to turn to the private sector and find ways to develop innovative financial products to fund this fiscal nightmare tied to ADRD in the years ahead.[38]

This chapter is central to the purpose of the book.

It acknowledges the *precedent set* with J. P. Morgan and the U.K. seeking to find new ways to finance ADRD and here, that action is extended by introducing two new financial products for investment banking firms to give thoughtful consideration for development. They are: 1) an Alzheimer's Disease Funding Note (ADFN) and 2) a Nutrition Certificate (NC).

States' Master Pool of Funds.

To ensure the legal and financial integrity of the two innovative financial products contemplated here, it is critical each state establishes an ADFN and NC pool of funds to support the offering of such new financial products to the investing public. It is thought that the pool would draw funds annually by a set percent established by law enacted in each state and taken from the following sources:

> * State lottery.
> * Cigarette tax revenue stream.
> * Gasoline tax.
> * Casino royalties.
> * Racetrack income.
> * Tax deductible donations from the private sector.

It is understood that states would not issue a separate obligation against the pool's assets. State law would prohibit the leveraging of the pool's deposits in any way whatsoever. That is to say the pool would

---

[38]   Pennsylvania State Plan on Alzheimer's Disease and Related Disorders. Recommendation No. 2. February 7, 2014.

be prohibited from engaging in futures, options, swaps and derivative products trading. Investment of the pool's funds would be limited to the purchase of bank and employee credit union certificates of deposit; and United States debt obligations such as: 1) Treasury Bills, 2) Treasury Notes and 3) Treasury Bonds. Each state's ADFN-NC Funding Pool would operate under the direction and supervision of each state's 'State Treasurer' or 'Comptroller.'

Alzheimer's Disease Funding Note.

The ADFN being proposed would be structured much like a state issued municipal bond with maturing dates of: 1) one year, 2) five and ten years and 3) twenty-five years.[39] To be competitive in the marketplace, the ADFN would pay one percent more than a corresponding federal debt obligation and the income would be free from federal and state tax obligations. These 'Notes' would be rated by such organizations as Moody's and Standard and Poor's and be suitable for investment made by trusts, profit sharing plans and state employee pension plans.

The issuance of ADFNs face value should not exceed the following amounts: 1) one year issues – one hundred percent liquid, 2) five and ten year denominations – five times the pool's assets and 3) twenty-five year obligations – ten times the pool's assets.

Proceeds from sale of ADFNs would be used to make subsidy support payments to CoEs and DPCs. Allocations of funds would be determined by the states and articulated in state law.

Nutrition Certificates.

Because food prices tend to adjust (usually upward) annually, the offering of NCs would be limited to one year obligations of the state.

---

[39] Reilly, Frank K. and Brown, Keith C. *Investment Analysis and Portfolio Management*. South-Western CENGAGE Learning, 2012, pp. 591-594 and 604.

Their structure would look much like that of a bank or credit union certificate of deposit, tax free (federal and state) interest bearing instrument with a one year claim on the pool's assets. The proceeds from the purchase and sale of NCs would be used to make food subsidy payments to CoEs, thereby reducing monthly costs to AD patients' DPC.

This is a grand opportunity for private organizations to partnership with the public sector and seek innovative ways to achieve some immediate (short-term) financial relief to CoEs and PDCs. Anchored to these two products are methodologies which provide for intermediate and long-term financial burdens as well.

The Marketplace.

With these innovative financial products, a new marketplace will emerge. This vehicle will allow for the free flow of funds of invested capital to move from one location to another. For example, should a particular state be in a need of funds, the marketplace will shift those funds from an overfunded location thereby bringing equilibrium to the entire infrastructure.

Conceptually, an ADFN would be expressed as: Name of the State – ADFN for Nonprofit (state) and (name of the CoE). There would be a coupon, maturity date, face amount and market value calculated by commonly understood and accepted methods of mark-to-the-market. The same would hold true for NCs. Their expression would be near the same. [40]

---

[40] Illustration Purposes Only: See Vanguard Municipal Bond Funds Statement of Net Assets (unaudited) As of: April 30, 2015, pp. 1 and 31.

The Marketplace

CHAPTER SEVEN

TAX REFORM

Governments last as long as the under-taxed can defend themselves against the over-taxed.

-Bernard Berenson

Hours worked go unpaid.

It is estimated that 17 billion hours of unpaid care are expended annually in the taking care of people stricken with AD by family members and friends.[41] At the current federal minimum wage rate of $7.25 an hour, this amounts to over $123 billion of lost income to the United States' economy each year. This is a shameful statistic for the richest, most powerful nation on the earth – and something should be done about it now!

Categories of Caregivers.

Here, three categories of caregivers to AD patients are identified. They are: 1) Caregiver, 2) Primary Caregiver and 3) Designated Primary Caregiver.

---

[41]   Lankford, Kimberly. <u>Planning for Alzheimer's.</u> *Kiplinger's Personal Finance.* April 2013.

For the most part, *Caregivers* are family members who go unpaid and provide daily assisted living to a family member stricken with AD. At a minimum, duties include: 1) feeding, 2) bathing, 3) dressing and 4) assistance with personal hygiene. Caregivers are also professionally licensed persons who come to a patient's residence daily, and provides like care for an AD patient. These Caregivers are paid – usually by the family, but there are instances where outside funding is available.

The *Primary Caregiver* is typically the spouse or nearest of kin who takes chief responsibility for the AD patient's well-being. It is a new term carved out in this text. It is best explained as in those instances where an AD patient is left single without a close blood family member, or legally adopted family member. The *Primary Caregiver* could be a person appointed to the position by a Court of Law. That person would be responsible for the safety, care and well-being of the AD patient.

Designated Primary Caregiver Program.

Designated Primary Caregiver is a new term introduced here in this chapter of the book. It is an official designation recognized by federal and state governments as having the ability to receive various forms of financial compensation and relief associated with their duties and responsibilities caring for an AD patient. The *Designated Primary Caregiver Program* might work something like this.

A Primary Caregiver would make application to Medicare and Medicaid Services which operates within the U.S. Department of Health and Human Services (HHS) to become officially recognized by that agency as the Designated Primary Giver for an AD patient. The formal application would include the following information:

* Name of the Designated Primary Caregiver (DPC) to include their Social Security Number.
* The legal address and telephone number of the DPC.

* Name and Social Security Number of the AD patient.
* Name and EIN of the CoE where the AD patient resides.
* A brief description of the AD patient's condition would be explained by a licensed qualifying medical physician.
* The application would be acknowledged by both the CoE and the attending medical doctor to the AD patient.
* An alternate DPC needs to be identified in the event the DPC precedes the AD patient in death.

This federal program will integrate easily with those states which have enacted Caregiver programs.[42]

Waste, Fraud and Abuse.

To help manage unintended consequences associated with the program, a number of safeguards would be put in place to avert waste, fraud and abuse.

First, only one person can be a DPC per AD patient. Second, the providing of social security numbers for persons and EINs for CoEs will provide a tracking system, an 'audit trail' capability to safeguard against criminal activity. When an AD patient dies, there would be an automatic notification to HHS that this event has occurred and benefits associated with the program would then cease.

It is contemplated this application and approval process would be timely and not be a lengthy, drawn out procedure. It would be expected that a sixty (60) day turnaround would be the maximum length of time for approval. Once a person has been recognized by HHS as a DPC, that person would be issued an identification card, much similar to a social security card in nature. The card will automatically expire upon the death of the AD patient.

Two special features would be associated with the card. First, DPC cardholders would receive annually a booklet containing

---

[42] The CARE Act; or Pennsylvania House Bill 1329.

fifty-two (52) coupons worth $100.00 each. These coupons would be able to be used at supermarkets to help with the cost of weekly purchases of groceries. They could be applied to food stuffs only and not tobacco substances, magazines or like paraphernalia. They could only be applied to what is commonly understood to be eatable food items. Second, for those companies who would elect to participate in the DPC program, cardholders would present their identification card at the time of purchase and would be given a ten percent (10%) discount on their total items bought. Tobacco and alcohol related products would be excluded.

A final recommended benefit for DPC cardholders would be a $2,000.00 income tax credit annually. This would provide direct monetary relief that is so much needed by caregivers of AD patients.

Centers of Excellence for Alzheimer's Disease.

These institutions provide the physical plant and trained personnel who care for AD patients who are no longer able to care for themselves or are at such a stage in the progression of the disease, that their PCG can no longer provide the care needed for the AD patient's safety and overall well-being.

As mentioned earlier, these organizations are sometimes funded by the states in which they reside; others operate as profit or non-profit institutions. In all cases, the buildings and grounds are in constant need of care and upkeep. The staff to care for AD patients is quite labor intensive. These factors combined, are extremely costly.

It is essential that new ways be explored to provide some financial relief to these institutions in order to contain costs, otherwise, the states' AD programs will fail and the federal government is not in a position to bailout this looming medical disaster waiting to happen.[43]

As a first step, the Internal Revenue Service (IRS) which operates under the U.S. Treasury Department has *Research and*

---

[43] Pennsylvania State Plan on Alzheimer's Disease and Related Disorders. Recommendation No. 4. February 7, 2014.

Experimentation Tax Credit or R&D Tax Credit, under IRS Code section 41 for companies that incur R&D costs in the United States. Many AD patients who are cared for at CoEs are indeed a part of living – ongoing research. Whether or not these activities would qualify for such tax credit is certainly worth exploring.

Where the building operation of a CoE might be subject to property tax obligations, community leaders, operators of CoEs and local government officials should come together and explore ways to either give some relief to those property tax obligations or ideally, allow them to operate with no property tax obligation at all.

One final thought. To enhance voluntary financial contributions to states' Master Pool of Funds, allow for those donations not only to be a state tax deductible item, but deductible with federal income tax obligations as well – with one caveat; rather than a 100% tax write-off, allow for a $125% write-off.

That is to say, if a person donated $1,000.00 to the AD Master Pool of Funds, rather than the deduction being $1,000.00, it would be $1,250.00. This would appeal especially to high net worth individuals who would be persuaded to favor such cause as AD over another.

This is not a panacea, or financial cure-all for funding the financial debacle associated with AD. At least it starts the debate and gets ideas in motion among industry professionals and lawmakers.

CHAPTER EIGHT

CONCLUSION

New opinions are always suspected, and usually opposed without any other reason but because they are not already common.

-John Locke (1632-1704)

"Doubt is an incitement to research, and Research is the Way which leads to Knowledge."[44]

Major pharmaceutical companies provide leadership in developing cutting edge technology to treat ADRD. Merck is one of those companies. A message from the company's board reads:

"Merck's vision is to help lead the world to a healthier future. Through our continuing commitment to scientific excellence and innovation in all aspects of our business, we aspire to create long-term value for society and all our shareholders."[45]

---

[44] David-Neel, Alexandra and Lama Yongden. *The Secret Oral Teachings in Tibetan Buddhist Sects.* San Francisco: City Light Books, 1967, p. 15.

[45] Harrison, Jr., William B. Chair, Committee on Governance, Public Policy and Corporate responsibility. Merck, July 2014.

Pfizer, another leading pharmaceutical – their mission statement says:

> "The mission of Pfizer's office of Independent Grants for Learning & Change, (IGL&C), formerly Medical Education Group (MEG), is to partner with the global healthcare community to improve patient outcomes in areas of mutual interest through support of measurable learning and change strategies."[46]

According to a recent Iowa State University study, certain proteins may slow the devastating memory loss caused by Alzheimer's disease. The report "found evidence that an elevated presence of a protein called neuronal pentraxin-2 may slow cognitive decline and reduce brain atrophy in people with Alzheimer's disease."[47]

"Researchers at the University of Virginia School of Medicine have discovered the brain is directly connected to the immune system by previously unknown vessels."[48] This discovery "will fundamentally change the way people look at the central nervous system's relationship with the human system."[49] The "discovery of these new vessels has enormous implications for every neurological disease with an immune component, from Alzheimer's to multiple sclerosis."[50]

Research and clinical trials are long-term strategies designed to eventually win the battle against ADRD. The works of major pharmaceutical companies and universities to seek lasting solutions to this devastating disease (ADRD) are noble. The problem is money and time.

The "latest estimate of the costs of drug development is $2.6 billion, according to the Tufts Center for the Study of Drug

---

[46] IGLC Mission Statement-Pfizer.

[47] Brown, Meg. Proteins may slow memory loss in people with Alzheimer's. Iowa State University College of Human Resources, May 21, 2015.

[48] Greenberg, Alissa. Game-Changing Discovery Links the Brain and the Immune System. Health Neuroscience, June 3, 2015.

[49] Ibid.

[50] Ibid.

Development."[51] "Lengthy clinical trials are required by the FDA in order to get a drug approved for marketing in the U.S. These trials can take as long as 11 years."[52]

What is needed right now are a number of short-term solutions to give immediate financial relief to caregivers of people stricken with ADRD and the CoEs who later provide for their well-being. In essence, that's what this book is about.

Nearly all 50 states are ill-prepared to effectively finance and administer an ADRD program. Equally, many lawmakers are unaware of their states financial condition and the financial obligations that go with the development and implementation of an ADRD program. Much of the public is not knowledgeable of this impending financial disaster coupled to ADRD. Investment bankers and interested law firms need to come forth, and bring ideas to the table for legislatures to consider in solving this looming medical problem.

Insurance companies who intend to offer medical coverage to the public need to develop more diversified products that can adequately meet the current financial shortfalls connected with ADRD. At the same time, those providers must look to the future and design medical insurance policies that have long range effects for the next generation.

Innovative financial products such as ADFNs and NCs are critical in meeting today's financial demands placed on society by ADRD. Without forward looking products such as these, the strains placed on the nation's citizenry are overwhelming.

Tax reform is essential in meeting the needs of all caregivers today. Many families are in dire financial straits because a family member has been stricken with AD. Time is not on lawmaker's side. Programs to provide for financial relief to ADRD families and CoEs must be designed now.

---

[51] Howard, Paul and Feyman, Yevgenly. The True Cost of Costly Drug Development.US News and World Report, May 20,2015

[52] Ibid.

EPILOGUE

Righteousness makes a nation great.
Proverbs 14:34[53]

Forward looking political leaders make great nations. They view their central role as having an ethical duty and moral responsibility for the safety and well-being of their citizenry. Today, Alzheimer's disease and related disorders are testing the courage of nations' leaders to exercise those duties and responsibilities not only for their countries' well-being, but for their very survival.

A Global Pandemic.

ADRD is not just a United States problem. Worldwide, 35.6 million people have dementia, of which 24.9 million have AD.[54] The World Health Organization reports "every year, there are 7.7 million new cases of people with the disease."[55] Clearly, ADRD is an international epidemic.[56]

---

[53] Stern, David H. *Complete Jewish Bible.* Jerusalem: Jewish New Testament Publications, Inc., 2012, p. 962.
[54] World Health Organization. Fact Sheet No. 362; 2012:2.
[55] World Health Organization. Fact Sheet No. 362; 2012:3, p. 1.
[56] World Health Organization. Fact Sheet No. 362; 2012:1.

Getting into a 'Crisis Action' mode.

On October 10, 2012, the National Institute on Aging announced a "new, publicly available database seeking to capture the full spectrum of current Alzheimer's disease research, investments and resources – both in the U.S. and internationally."[57] This resource will help manage overlapping research efforts and better make available a condensed set of findings and applications for continued study and work. These are wonderful breakthroughs and offer hope to those who, until now, had no hope.

Setting aside innovative financial products and meaningful tax reform, the ultimate solution to the Alzheimer's disease global epidemic hinges on the answer to one question.

The medical industry and lawmakers need to address a question essential to the looming financial disaster associated with Alzheimer's disease, and that question is this. What is the risk-reward; the trade-offs, between the industry's current infrastructure and the determination and redirection of resources to seek a cure for Alzheimer's disease? Until a transparent debate takes place about this and an agreed upon consensus is arrived at, this issue will remain unresolved and the world population will continue to be plagued by this horrid disease.

---

[57] National Institute on Aging. New database aims to capture international Alzheimer's disease research efforts. October 10, 2012.

APPENDICES

Appendix A – List of Organizations that Provide Information about ADRD.

Appendix B – Typical AD patient's Daily Schedule at a Center of Excellence for Alzheimer's. Disease.

Appendix C – Film Reference: *Still Alice.*

Appendix D – The National Alzheimer's Project Act of 2011.

APPENDICES

List of Organizations that Provide Information about ADRD.

AARP
601 E Street, NW
Washington, DC 20049

(888) 687-2277

Alzheimer's Association
225 N. Michigan Avenue
Floor 17
Chicago, IL 60601

(800) 272-3900

US Department of Health and Human Services
Alzheimer's Disease Education and Referral Center
Bldg. 31, Room 5C27
31 Center Drive, MSC 2292
Bethesda, MD 20892

(800) 438-4380

Alzheimer's Foundation of America
322 Eighth Avenue
7th Floor
New York, NY 10001

(866) 232-8484

www.caregiver.org/family-care-navigator

Typical ADRD Patient's Daily Schedule at a Center of Excellence for AD.

7:30 – 8:45 Breakfast
8:45 – 9:00 Life Skills
9:00 – 9:15 Meet and Greet
9:15 – 9:30 Reminiscence Group
9:30 – 10:00 Exercise Group
10:00 – 10:30 Snack & Socializing
10:30 – 10:45 Storytelling
10:45 – 11:00 Sing–along
11:00 – 11:30 Lunch Preparation/Therapeutic Chores
11:30 – 12:00 Pre–lunch Social
12:00 – 1:00 Lunch
1:00 – 1:30 Quiet Time/Gathering
1:30 – 2:00 Dual Programming/Sensory Stimulation
2:00 – 2:15 Escorting
2:15 – 2:45 Snack & Socializing
2:45 – 3:00 Sing–along
3:00 – 3:15 Exercise Group
3:15 – 3:30 Drink Break
3:30 – 3:45 Word Game
3:45 – 4:00 Afternoon Stretch
4:00 – 4:30 Group Project/Craft/Active Game

4:30 - 5:00 Supper Preparation/Therapeutic Chores
5:00 - 5:30 Pre-Supper Social
5:30 - 6:45 Supper
6:45 - 7:00 Reminiscence/Word Games/Current Events
7:00 - 7:15 Evening Stretch
7:15 - 7:30 Sing-along
7:30 - 7:45 Snack & Socializing
7:45 - 8:00 Music Video
8:00 - 9:00 Preparation for bedtime

* Special programs including pet visits, musical performances, intergenerational programs, craft and cooking groups, individual manicures and individual reading are offered on a monthly basis. Devotions are held twice a week. Regular Bible study is offered by most all CoEs. Many organizations have a full-time, interdenominational, Chaplain on staff and devotions are typically held on Sunday mornings.

Appendix C

Film Reference

Glatzer, Richard and Westmoreland, Wash. **Still Alice**. DVD
Video. Sony Pictures Classics. PG-13. 2015.

Appendix D

PUBLIC LAW 111-375-JAN. 4, 2011

NATIONAL ALZHEIMER'S PROJECT ACT

GLOSSARY OF SELECTED TERMS

AARP – formerly known as the American Association of Retired Persons, AARP is the nation's leading organization for people age fifty and older. Founded in 1958 by retired educator Dr. Ethel Percy Andrus, it is a nonprofit, nonpartisan association with a membership of 40 million. Its mission is to promote the welfare of senior citizens.

Alzheimer's Association – works on a global, national and local level to enhance care and support for all those affected by Alzheimer's and other dementias. Its mission is to eliminate Alzheimer's disease through the advancement of research; to provide and enhance care and support for all affected; and to reduce the risk of dementia through the promotion of brain health.

Alzheimer's disease – is characterized by loss of memory to the point so severe that it interferes with a person's activities associated with daily living. Early signs common to Alzheimer's disease are the inability to remember even simple things. Reasoning is visibly impaired and there's little interest in planning.

Alzheimer's Disease Funding Note – is a newly contemplated financial instrument whereby the proceeds from sales of such securities are used to fund various state programs involved with the mechanics and workings of states' ADRD programs.

Alzheimer's Disease International – was founded in 1984 to help fight Alzheimer's disease, first diagnosed in 1906. It is the umbrella organization of more than 80 Alzheimer's associations around the world.

Centers of Excellence for Alzheimer's Disease – also called Alzheimer's Disease Assistance Centers, healthcare facilities; these are profit and nonprofit organizations that have a physical location that provides full-time professional care for those afflicted with Alzheimer's disease.

Gross Domestic Product – the total value of goods produced and services provided in a country during one year.

National Alzheimer's Project Act of 2010 – (Public Law 111-375), passed unanimously by Congress in December 2010 and signed into law by President Barack Obama in January 2011. This legislation provided for the creation of a national strategic plan to address the rapidly escalating Alzheimer's disease crisis and the coordination of Alzheimer's disease efforts across the federal government.

Nutrition Certificate – is a newly contemplated financial instrument whereby the proceeds from the sale of such securities are used to help reduce the cost of food products used by CoEs in the care of their ADRD patients.

Tax Reform – refers to Chapter Seven of the text and sets forth a number of ideas and suggestions for lawmakers to consider in reforming federal and state tax codes in order to give some financial relief to caregivers and facility providers of those afflicted with Alzheimer's disease.

The United Nations – is an intergovernmental organization established on October 24, 1945 to promote international cooperation. It was a replacement for the ineffective League of Nations. The organization was created following the Second World War to prevent another such horrific conflict.

U.S. Department of Health and Human Services – administers federal programs dealing with public health, welfare, and income security; created in 1979 from the reorganized Department of Health, Education and Welfare. Abbreviation: HHS.

BIBLIOGRAPHY

Alzheimer's Association. Alzheimer's Disease Facts and Figures 2015.

American Psychiatric Association. *Diagnostic and Statistical Manual of Mental Disorders.* 5th. Arlington, VA: American Psychiatric Publishing; 2013:section 2.

Brown, Meg. Proteins may slow memory loss in people with Alzheimer's. Iowa State University College of Human Resources. May 21, 2015.

David-Neel, Alexandra and Lama Yongden. *The Secret Oral Teachings in Tibetan Buddhist Sects.* San Francisco: City Lights Books, 1967.

de la Merced, Michael and Abelson, Reed. Cigna Rejects an Overture From Anthem. *The New York Times.* Section B1. Monday, June 22, 2015.

Forbes, Steve. The Constitution Does It Matter Anymore? *Forbes.* July 20, 2015.

Glatzer, Richard and Westmorland, Wash. *Still Alice.* Killer Films. DVD. December 5, 2014.

Goodnough, Abby. Barely Meeting a Law It Hoped to Transcend. *The New York Times.* Friday, June 5, 2015.

Greenberg, Alissa. Game-Changing Discovery Links the Brain and the Immune System. Health Neuroscience. June 3, 2015.

Harrison, Jr., William B. Chair, Committee on Governance, Public Policy and Corporate Responsibility, Merck, July 2014.

Haskins, Ron. The federal debt is worse than you think. Washington: *The Brookings Institution.* April 8, 2015.

Hms.harvard.edu.

Hoffman, David. Alzheimer's Disease Caregiver Support Initiative. *Advisory Council on Alzheimer's Research, Care, and Services.* US Department of Health and Human Services, 200 Independence Avenue, SW, Washington, DC. July 27, 2015.

Howard, Paul and Feyman, Yevgenly. The True Cost of Costly Drug Development. US News and World Report. May 20, 2015.

http://youtu.be/LL Gq7She-Y

IGLC Mission Statement. Pfizer.

Internal Revenue Service section 41.

Kandel, Eric R., Schwartz, James H., Jessell, Thomas M., Siegelbaum, Steven A. and Hudspeth, A. J. (ed.). *Principles of Neural Science.* New York: McGraw-Medical, 2013.

Kiplinger's Retirement Report. Don't Get Trapped By Medicare Rules. May 2015.

Lankford, Kimberly. Planning for Alzheimer's. *Kiplinger's Personal Finance.* April 2013.

Morens, David M. and Fauci, Anthony S. The 1918 Influenza Pandemic: Insights for the 21st Century. Oxford: The Journal of Infectious Diseases. Volume 195, Issue 7, pp. 1018-1028, 2007.

National Institute of Health. *NIH-supported study finds U.S. dementia care costs as high as $215 billion in 2010*; April 3, 2013.

National Institute on Aging. Fact Sheet; 2014:1.

National Institute on Aging. New database aims to capture international Alzheimer's disease research efforts. October 10, 2012.

Neurology: 2014; 82(12): 1045-50.

Nolen-Hoeksema, Susan, Fredrickson, Barbara L., Loftus, Geoffrey R. and Lutz, Christel. *Atkinson & Hilgard's:Introduction to Psychology*. Andover: Cengage Learning, 2014.

Pearsall, Judy. *The Concise Oxford Dictionary*. Oxford: Oxford University Press, 1999.

Pennsylvania State Plan on Alzheimer's Disease and Related Disorders. Seven Recommendations. February 7, 2014.

Reilly, Frank K. and Brown, Keith C. *Investment Analysis and Portfolio Management*. South-Western CENGAGE Learning, 2012.

Reinhard, Susan C., Feinberg, Lynn Friss, Choula, Rita and Houser, Ari. Valuing the Invaluable:2015 Update. AARP Public Policy Institute, July 2015.

Sorkin, Andrew Ross. Health Care Law Spurs Merger Talks for Insurers. *The New York Times*. Business Section. June 22, 2015.

Stern, David H. *Complete Jewish Bible.* Jerusalem: Jewish New Testament Publications, Inc., 2012.

The CARE Act; or Pennsylvania House Bill 1329.

The Kiplinger Letter. Vol. 92, No. 31. July 31, 2015.

The National Alzheimer's Project Act (Public Law 111-375).

Vanguard Municipal Bond Funds Statement of Net Assets (unaudited) as of: April 30, 2015.

WebMD Medical Reference. SOURCE: Alzheimer's Association. Reviewed by: Neil Lava, M.D. on: July 10, 2014.

Wells, Samuel. Dementia and resurrection. London: Christian Century, April 1, 2015.

World Health Organization. Fact Sheets No. 362; 2012:1-3

www.truthinaccounting.org

ABOUT THE AUTHOR

B udd Hallberg started his career in 1966 as an investment banker; first with Francis I. DuPont & Company, then Dominick & Dominick, Inc., and later Hornblower & Weeks-Hemphill, Noyes, Inc. He was a member of the New York Coffee, Sugar and Cocoa Exchange, the New York Cotton Exchange and the New York Mercantile Exchange.

In 1976 Hallberg joined the U.S. Commodity Futures Trading Commission (CFTC) in Washington, DC. In 1979 the CFTC awarded him the federal government's Meritorious Service Award. He was appointed a Director of the agency that same year. From 1985 until his retirement in 2007 Hallberg was the President of SCAN Management Inc., a management consulting firm located in Gettysburg, Pennsylvania. He is a member of the Chartered Financial Analyst Society of Philadelphia.

In 1965 Hallberg was appointed a Reserve Commissioned Officer in the Army of the United States. He is a graduate of the Command and General Staff College of the United States Army. Hallberg is the recipient of the Meritorious Service Medal and the Army Commendation Medal with two Oak Leaf Clusters. He retired from the United States Army at the rank of Lieutenant Colonel in 2002.

In 2004 Hallberg became an adjunct faculty member of the HACC-Gettysburg campus and teaches Introduction to Philosophy and Logic. He is a member of the HACC Foundation Board of Directors.

Hallberg is a member of the AARP Citizen Advocate Team in Harrisburg, Pennsylvania. He works specifically in the area of

Alzheimer's disease and related disorders. Hallberg volunteers time each week at a Center of Excellence for AD residents in Hanover, Pennsylvania. He is a former caregiver. His wife died of cancer in January 2011.

INDEX

www.ingramcontent.com/pod-product-compliance
Lightning Source LLC
Chambersburg PA
CBHW020902310526
45786CB00018B/1550